Maryem Ferjani

Antibiotic resistance in childhood urinary tract infections

Maryem Ferjani

Antibiotic resistance in childhood urinary tract infections

ScienciaScripts

This book is a translation from the original published under ISBN 978-620-3-45823-7.

Publisher:
Sciencia Scripts
is a trademark of
Dodo Books Indian Ocean Ltd. and OmniScriptum S.R.L publishing group

120 High Road, East Finchley, London, N2 9ED, United Kingdom
Str. Armeneasca 28/1, office 1, Chisinau MD-2012, Republic of Moldova, Europe
Printed at: see last page
ISBN: 978-620-6-07129-7

INTRODUCTION

Many epidemiological studies attempt to identify risk or protective factors for a given disease, in order to implement preventive measures and/or adapt therapeutic strategies. Logistic regression is one of the most widely used multivariate statistical analyses in epidemiology. It is a modelling technique which aims to predict and explain the values of a binary categorical variable Y (predictor variable, explained variable, dependent variable, class attribute, endogenous variable) from a collection of continuous or binary variables X (predictor variables, explanatory variables, independent variables, descriptors, exogenous variables) (1) . It provides a powerful means of quantifying the association between a disease under study and each of the factors influencing it, taking into account the simultaneous effect of other factors. This tool would make a major contribution to the study of antibiotic resistance factors in childhood urinary tract infections (UTIs).UTIs are common and are a source of renal scarring, leading in the long term to nephron reduction, chronic renal failure and hypertension (2-4). Appropriate early empirical antibiotic treatment is crucial to prevent sequelae (5). Empirical treatment must be based on knowledge of the epidemiology of antibiotic resistance, to ensure rapid efficacy and cure (6,7). In recent years, several antibiotic-resistant strains have emerged worldwide, leading experts to adapt their therapeutic strategies. Indeed, the growing antibiotic resistance of bacteria involved in UTIs, especially for commonly used antibiotics, limits the choice of antibiotics, hence the importance of bacteriological documentation and the choice of appropriate antibiotic therapy (6). In our country, data on the profile of urinary tract infection germs and their resistance are updated annually on the national network for monitoring antibiotic resistance, but the risk factors for antibiotic resistance have not previously been studied. We need to study the profile of strains observed, as well as the risk factors associated with these resistances, in order to update our therapeutic management. Indeed, it is essential to offer optimized management of patients with UTIs, given the changing epidemiology of antibiotic resistance. To what extent can logistic regression control possible confounding biases among variables, and highlight independent risk factors for antibiotic resistance in children? The aim of our work was to determine the risk factors associated with UTIs caused by strains of extended-spectrum betalactamase (ESBL)-producing Enterobacteriaceae in children.

METHODS

I. TYPE OF STUDY

This was a cross-sectional etiological study of a series of children admitted for UTI.

1. Patients :

1.1. Inclusion criteria:

We included all children admitted for suspected UTI to the pediatric nephrology department whose infection was confirmed by a positive urine cytobacteriological examination (UCE) culture from January to September 2020. We included only the first positive urine culture obtained per patient on admission and positive aerobic bacterial cultures.

1.2. Non-inclusion criteria:

We did not include in the study children with a positive ECBU but no symptoms suggestive of UTI. These were asymptomatic bacteriuria, and the ECBU was requested prior to a radiological examination or therapeutic procedure. We did not include fungal UTIs.

1.3. Exclusion criteria :

We excluded patients with a culture that showed three or more germs, a culture that found a germ but at an insignificant rate according to the sampling method, or a culture that showed the outbreak of a germ considered contaminating. We also excluded patients with a documented UTI who were over 18 years of age.

2. COURSE OF THE STUDY

All files were reviewed by a single examiner. We collected data relating to the interview, clinical and para-clinical examinations carried out during hospitalization. All information was recorded on a chart (Appendix 1).

3. Questioning data

We have collected the following data:

-Reason for hospitalization

-Age

-The sex

-Previous hospitalizations

-Presence or absence of immune deficiency

-Known uropathy and its nature

-Vulvitis

-History of UTI

-History of urological surgery

-History of invasive imaging of the urinary tract: urodynamic testing (UDT), retrograde urethrocystography (RUC)

-Antibiotic therapy within the last 3 or 6 months

4. Clinical examination data

We recorded the data from the clinical examination on admission, as shown in Appendix 1.

5. Additional test data :

Reports of other complementary examinations already carried out were noted on the canvas. These examinations included :

5.1. Renal function:

We recorded the different creatinine values of the patients and calculated creatinine clearance according to the Schwartz formula:

*Creatinine clearance=36.5*height (cm)/blood creatinine (umol/L)*

5.2. Cytobacteriological examination of urine:

A first approach was to examine urine by dipstick for nitrites and leukocytes.

The strip detects the presence of leukocytes through the leukocyte esterase reaction, and bacteria through the detection of nitrites. In the presence of Gram-negative fermenting bacteria (enterobacteria), nitrates present in the bladder are transformed into nitrites.If leukocyturia and nitrites are both negative, the diagnosis of UTI is unlikely (false negative < 10%). However, if only one parameter is positive, we recommend ECBU (8). are not reliable before the age of one month, and that an ECBU was systematically requested (9).

Diagnosis of UTI is based on the results of both direct examination and quantitative culture: bacteriuria greater than 10^5 CFU/ml if midstream urine sample is taken, with or without pathological leukocyturia (greater than 10^4 leukocytes/ml). Culture and germ identification take 24 hours, and antibiotic susceptibility testing 36 to 48 hours. The method of urine collection was taken into account when interpreting the culture according to the recommendations of Rémic 2018 (10). Each urine sample received at the laboratory underwent a cytobacteriological examination comprising:

• A direct examination to assess leukocyturia and other figurative elements in the urine (red blood cells, crystals), performed under a light microscope with a 40° objective.

• Bacterial culture by counting the number and type of germs.

• An antibiotic susceptibility test to determine the sensitivity of isolated bacteria to antibiotics.

Bacteria were identified on the basis of conventional morphological, cultural and biochemical characteristics, using both manual and automated methods (VITEK 2 Compact, bioMérieux®).Antibiotic susceptibility testing was carried out using the Muller Hinton agar disk diffusion technique, and interpretation was made according to the standards of the Comité de l'antibiogramme de la Société française de microbiologie (CA-SFM).Third-generation cephalosporin-resistant (CIIIG) strains of ESBL-producing Enterobacteriaceae were systematically identified on the susceptibility test by the synergy test between a central disk of amoxicillin + clavulanic acid and disks of beta-lactam antibiotics (cefotaxime, ceftazidime, cefepime and aztreonam). The presence of ESBLs was noted by a "champagne cork" appearance. For CIIIG-resistant strains, and in the absence of the synergy image, the test was repeated, adding 250mg/l of cloxacillin to Mueller Hinton agar to inhibit any cephalosporinase and thus reveal any double synergy.Multi-resistant bacteria (MRB) include ESBL-producing Enterobacteriaceae, cephalosporinase-producing Enterobacteriaceae, etc. carbapenemase-producing enterobacteria, imipenem-resistant Pseudomonas aeruginosa, imipenem-resistant acinetobacter baumannii, methicillin-resistant satphylococcus aureus and vancomycin-resistant enterobacteria.mMinimum inhibitory concentrations (MICs) for ertapenem, imipenem and meropenem were determined using the bioMérieux® E-test method on MH agar whenever an isolated enterobacteria showed an inhibition diameter around the ertapenem disc < 25 mm. If carbapenemase production by these bacteria was suspected, a Carbapenem Inactivation Method (CIM) phenotypic test was performed.

The variables used in the present work were :

- Age: this discrete quantitative variable varied in our work between 0 and 18 years of age. This same variable was transformed into a qualitative ordinal variable by grouping four age groups in months

- Gender: this nominal qualitative variable had two categories in our work feminine and masculine.

-Previous hospitalization: this binary qualitative variable had two categories in our work, either yes or no, depending on the presence or absence of a previous hospitalization.

-Fever: this binary qualitative variable had two categories in our work, depending on whether or not the initial fever lasted more than 48 hours.

-Intermittent probes: this binary qualitative variable had two categories in our work, depending on whether the patient was on intermittent probes or not.

-Underlying uropathy: this binary qualitative variable had two categories in our work, depending on whether the child had underlying uroptahy or not.

-Recurrence of UTI: binary qualitative variable. It was defined by the occurrence of 2 or more episodes of UTI in the recurrence subgroup. It therefore comprised two categories, depending on whether or not UTIs had recurred in the past.

-Antibiotic therapy taken in the previous three months: this binary qualitative variable also had two categories in our work: yes, no, depending on the antibiotic taken. antibiotics in the three months preceding the episode of UTI considered in our study.

-Antibiotic prophylaxis: this binary qualitative variable also had two categories in our work, either yes or no, depending on whether or not antibiotic prophylaxis was taken. Finally, the dependent variable used in our work was the presence of an ESBL strain, which is a qualitative binary variable with two categories depending on the characteristic of the strain incriminated in the UTI: whether it is an ESBL strain or not.

III. STATISTICAL ANALYSIS :

1. Data entry and preparation for analysis :

Data were collected retrospectively from medical records. The information collected was treated confidentially. Data analysis in our work was carried out using SPSS ("Statistical Package for Social Sciences") version 26 and Microsoft Excel 2013 for graphics.

2. Descriptive analysis :

This was the first part of our study. It enabled us to describe the entire population concerned by UTIs. It included all children aged between 0 and 18. Only one quantitative variable was used: age. This was described by its mean. The other qualitative variables were described by percentages.

3. Etiological analysis :

3.1. Bi-variate analysis :

Comparisons between two categorical variables or the search for links between two categorical variables (two percentages) were carried out using Pearson's x2 test; and in the event of statistical significance but invalidity, using Fisher's exact test. Results are expressed in terms of significance (p-value) at a 5% risk of error. A p-value <0.05 means that the difference is significant.

Measures of association, including the crude Odds Ratio (ORb) and its 95% confidence interval (CI), were determined using simple binary logistic regression.

3.2. Multivariate analysis :

To determine the factors independently associated or not with the presence of antibiotic resistance, we ran a binary logistic regression model. The dependent variable was the presence or absence of an ESBL strain. The reference category chosen in the regression model was the presence of an ESBL strain. Only explanatory variables with a significance level "p" of less than 0.2 in the bivariate analysis were included in the multivariate analysis. The number of variables introduced was estimated so that for each explanatory variable we had at least five events of the least numerous modality of the dependent variable. The method used to introduce variables into the model was top-down (Wald stepwise)(11).

The significance level of the "Wald" test was used to determine whether each independent variable contributed significantly to the improvement of the logistic regression model. As in the bi-variate analysis, the significance level was $p<0.05$. For the final model, we have presented adjusted Odds Ratios (ORa) and their 95% CIs for the variables introduced in the regression model.

Goodness of fit was also verified by two tests:
- The pseudo R-two (Cox and Snell and Nagelkerke adjusted) was used to estimate the percentage variability of the dependent variable by the explanatory variables.

- The classification table was used to estimate the percentage of observations classified in one or other modality of the dependent variable, as predicted by the regression model.

The Hosmer-Lemeshow test was also used to validate the regression model.

IV. ETHICAL CONSIDERATIONS :

Confidentiality was respected during data processing. There were no conflicts of interest to declare.

V. BIBLIOGRAPHIC SEARCH :

This search was developed by selecting articles from PubMed, Science Directe, EM premium and Google Scholar using the following keywords: logistic regression, urinary tract infection, antibiotic resistance, child.

RESULTS

I. DESCRIPTIVE STUDY :

1. Clinical characteristics of the population :

A total of 100 episodes of bacteriologically confirmed urinary tract infections were included in the study. The 100 episodes involved 100 patients.

1.1. Gender :

There were 38 boys and 62 girls. The sex ratio of girls to boys was 0.6.

1.2. Age :

The average age of all patients was 59.7 months, with extremes ranging from 3 days to 17 years. The age distribution of our population is shown in Figure 1.

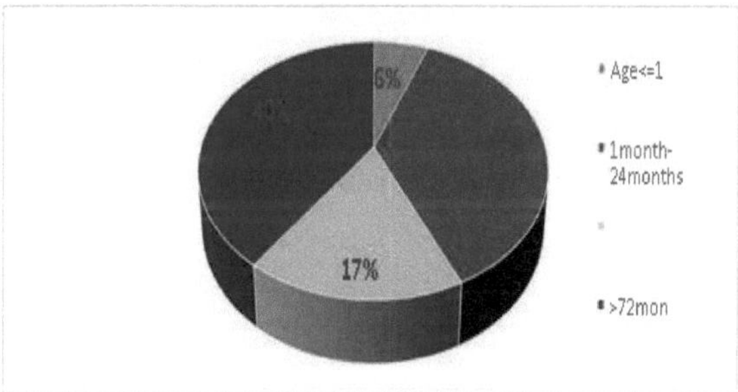

Figure 1: Patient distribution by age group

In newborns and infants, urinary tract infections mainly affected boys, while in children and older children, the female sex was most affected. The gender distribution was significant, with a p < 0.001 (Figure 2).

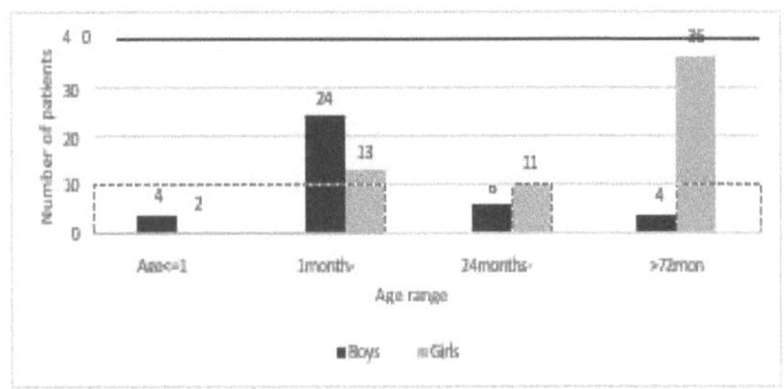

Figure 2: Distribution of urinary tract infections by patient gender and age group

1.3. Urine sampling technique :

The most commonly used collection technique was mid-jet collection, followed by collection via the urine collector (figure 3).

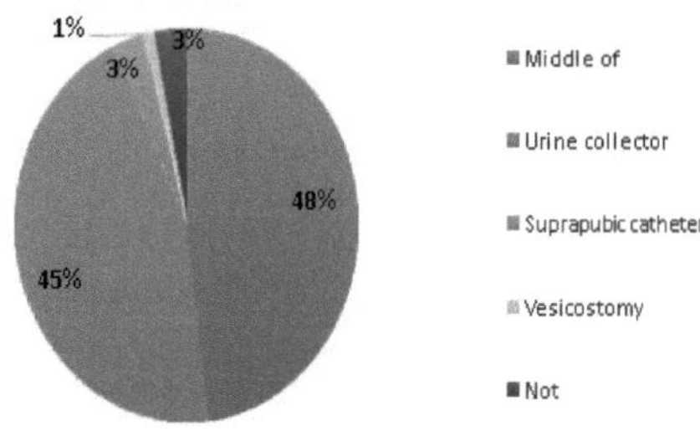

Figure 3: Urine sampling methods

2. Epidemiological profiles :

2.1. Germs involved :

Escherichia coli dominated the epidemiological profile (66%), followed by Klebsiella pneumonia (14%) and Pseudomonas aeruginosa (7%).Table I illustrates the epidemiological profile of our series.

Table I. Distribution of bacteria responsible for urinary tract infections in children

Germ	Percentage
Escherichia coli	66
Klebsiella pneumoniae	14
Pseudomonas aeruginosa	7
Proteus mirabilis	3
Acinetobacter baumannii	1
Klebsiella oxytoca	3
Enterococcus faecalis	2
Staphylococcus ludgensis	1
Citrobacter freundii	1
Morganella morganii	2
Total	100

2.2. Bacteriological profile by age :

Two bacteria dominated the UTI profile in newborns: Escherichia coli (50%) and Klebsiella pneumoniae (25%). In other age groups, Escherichia coli dominated the bacteriological profile, followed by Klebsiella pneumoniae in infants and Pseudomonas in children over 2 years of age (figure 4)

.

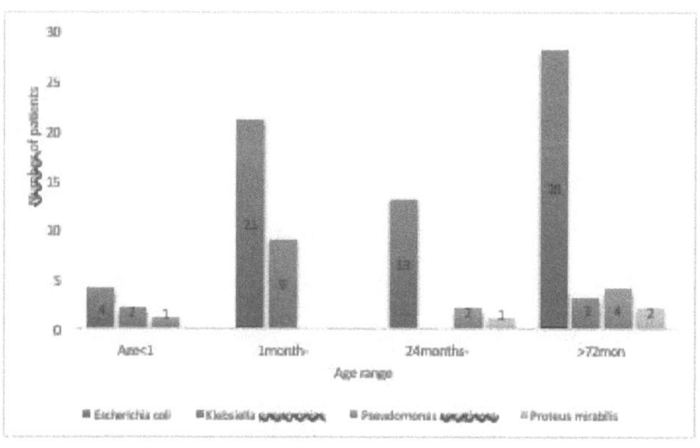

Figure 4: Distribution of bacterial species by age group

2.3. Bacteriological profile by sex :

In our study, the germ most frequently isolated in girls was Escherichia coli (71%). Similarly, the majority of boys had positive cultures for Escherichia coli (58%).

3. Global antibiotic susceptibility study :

Overall antibiotic sensitivity for all germs combined showed 39% resistance to amoxicillin-clavulanic acid; forty-eight percent to first-generation cephalosporins, forty-two percent to second-generation cephalosporins, thirty-nine percent resistance to cefixime, forty-one percent to cefotaxime, thirty-four percent to ceftazidime and 41% to trimetoprim-sulfametoxazole (TPM-SMX).Nitrofurantoin, fluoroquinolones and aminoglycosides were the most active molecules, with resistance rates of 9%, seventeen percent, eighteen percent and 5% respectively for nitrofurantoin, ciprofloxacin, gentamicin and amikacin (Figure 5).

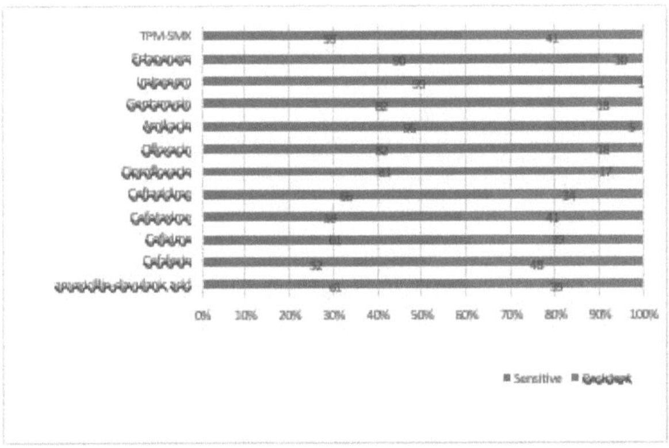

Figure 5: Resistance rates to the main antibiotics recommended for the
treatment of urinary tract infections in children

Escherichia coli were resistant to amoxicillin and clavulanic acid in 26% of cases, to cefixime and cefotaxime in 28.8%, to ceftazidime in 27.3% and to TPM- SMX in 12.5%. The resistance profile of Escherichia coli isolates is shown in figure 6.

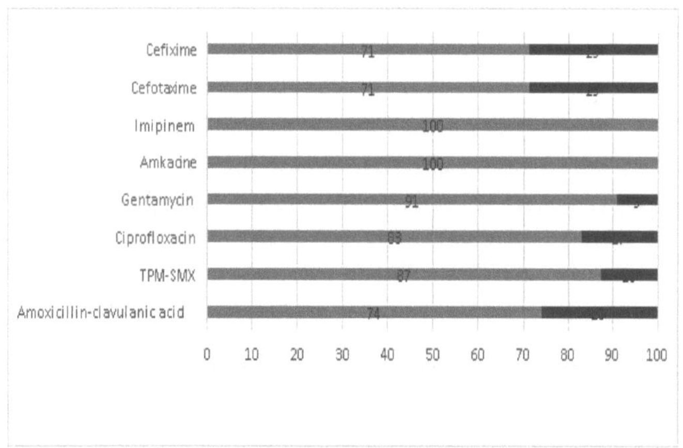

Figure 6. Resistance rates of Escherichia coli isolates to the various antibiotics tested

ESBL production among isolated Enterobacteriaceae was 29%, and BMR prevalence was 28%. The distribution of ESBL Enterobacteriaceae shows a clear predominance of Escherichia coli (65.5%), followed by Klebsiella pneumonia (34.5%). Carbapenem susceptibility testing revealed 10% resistance to ertapenem and only 1% to imipenem.

II. ANALYTICAL STUDY OFFACTORS OF ANTIBIOTIC RESISTANCE :

1. Univariate study:

1.1. Antibiotic susceptibility by age :

We studied antibiotic resistance in the different age groups: group 1 under 1 month (n=8), group 2 between 1 month and 24 months (n=36), group between 24 months and 72 months (n=16) and group 4 between 72 months and 18 years (n=40). We found a statistically significant difference between groups for amoxicillin-clavulanic acid and gentamycin, but no difference for ESBL strains (Table II).

Table II. Antibiotic susceptibility by age group

			Age<1mois	1-24mois	24-72mois	>72months	P
			n / %	n / %	n / %	n / %	
Amoxicillin-clavulanic acid	S	n	4	15	11	31	0.009
		%	50	41.7	68.8	77.5	
	R	n	4	21	5	9	
		%	50	58.3	31.3	22.5	
Cefuroxime	S	n	4	18	9	27	0.427
		%	50	50	56.3	67.5	
	R	n	4	18	7	13	
		%	50	50	43.8	32.5	
Cefixime	S	n	4	18	9	30	0.118
		%	50	50	56.3	75	
	R	n	4	18	7	10	
		%	50	50	43.8	25	
Cefotaxime	S	n	4	18	9	28	0.318
		%	50	50	56.3	70	
	R	n	4	18	7	12	
		%	50	50	43.8	30	
Ceftazidime	S	n	5	19	11	31	0.147
		%	62.5	52.8	68.8	77.5	
	R	n	3	17	5	9	
		%	37.5	47.2	31.3	22.5	
Imipenem	S	n	8	35	16	40	0.6
		%	100	97.2	100	100	
	R	n	0	1	0	0	
		%	0	2.8	0	0	
TPM-SMX	S	n	5	24	9	21	0.65
		%	62.5	66.7	56.3	52.5	
	R	n	3	12	7	19	
		%	37.5	33.3	43.8	47.5	
Amikacin	S	n	8	33	16	38	0.737
		%	100	91.7	100	95	
	R	n	0	3	0	2	
		%	0	8.7	0	5	
Gentamycin	S	n	6	25	13	38	0.017
		%	75	69.4	81.3	95	
	R	n	2	11	3	2	
		%	25	30.6	18.8	5	
ESBL	S	n	2	14	5	8	0.336
		%	25	38.9	31.8	20	
	R	n	6	22	11	32	
		%	75	61.1	68.8	80	
	YES						
	NO						

S : sensitive, R : resistant

1.2. Antibiotic susceptibility by sex :

We examined resistance by sex, the first group being girls (n=62) and the second boys (n=38). Resistance to was significantly higher with amoxicillin-clavulanic acid and gentamycin, but no difference was noted for ESBL strains (Table III).

Table III. Antibiotic susceptibility by sex

		Girls		Boys	
		n	%	n	%
Amoxicillin-clavulanic acid	S	45	72.6	16	42.1
	R	17	27.4	22	39
Cefuroxime	S	38	61.3	20	52.6
	R	24	38.7	18	47.4
Cefixime	S	41	66.1	20	52.6
	R	21	33.9	18	47.4
Cefotaxime	S	39	62.9	20	52.6
	R	23	37.1	18	47.4
Ceftazidime	S	43	69.4	23	60.5
	R	19	30.6	15	39.5
Imipenem	S	62	100	37	97.4
	R	0	0	1	2.6
TPM-SMX	S	38	61.3	21	55.5
	R	24	38.7	17	44.7
Amikacin	S	60	96.8	35	92.1
	R	2	3.2	3	7.9
Gentamycin	S	57	91.9	25	65.8
	R	5	8.1	13	34.2
ESBL	S	18	29	11	29
	R	44	61	27	61

S : sensitive R : resistant

1.3. Sensitivity according to recurrence of urinary tract infections :

We examined resistance in first-episode UTIs (n=22) and in recurrent UTIs (n=78). There was no statistically significant difference between the two groups for the different antibiotics (Table IV). The comparison of ESBL strains between the two groups did not reveal any statistically significant difference.

Table IV. Antibiotic susceptibility according to recurrence of urinary tract infections

		Premier épisode d'infection urinaire n %	Infections urinaires à répétition n %	p
Amoxicilline-acide clavulanique	S	13 59.1	48 61.5	1
	R	9 40.9	30 38.5	
Cefuroxime	S	16 72.7	42 53.8	0.145
	R	6 27.3	36 46.2	
Cefixime	S	17 77.3	44 56.4	0.088
	R	5 22.7	34 43.6	
Cefotaxime	S	16 72.7	43 55.1	0.152
	R	43 55.1	35 44.9	
Ceftazidime	S	18 81.8	48 61.5	0.125
	R	4 18.2	30 38.5	
Imipenème	S	22 100	77 98.7	1
	R	0 0	1 1.3	
TPM-SMX	S	17 77.3	42 53.8	0.054
	R	5 22.7	36 46.2	
Amikacine	S	22 100	73 93.6	0.583
	R	0 0	5 6.4	
Gentamycine	S	21 95.5	61 78.2	0.112
	R	1 4.5	17 21.8	
BLSE	OUI	3 13.6	26 33.4	0.109
	NON	19 86.4	52 66.6	

S :sensible, R :résistant

1.4. Antibiotic sensitivity according to fever duration :

Antibiotic resistance was analyzed by dividing patients into 2 groups: the first group of patients with fever <48 hours (n=68) and the second group with fever lasting more than 48 hours (n=32). There were no statistically significant differences between the two groups, either for the different antibiotics tested or for ESBL strains (Table V).

Table V. Antibiotic sensitivity according to fever duration

Fever <48Fever >48

Hours n %		Hours p n %	
S	39	22	
Amoxicillin-clavulanic acid	57.4	68.8	0.38
R	29	10	
42.6		31.3	
S	38	20	
Cefuroxime	55.9	62.5	0.665
R	30	12	
44.1		37.5	
S	41	20	
Cefixime	60.3	62.5	1
R	27	12	
39.7		37.5	
S	39	20	
Cefotaxime	57.4	62.5	0.668
R	29	12	
42.6		37.5	
S	46	20	
Ceftazidime	67.6	62.5	0.655
R	22	12	
32.4		37.5	
S	67	32	
Imipenem	98.5	100	1
R	1	0	
1.5		0	
S	38	21	
TPM-SMX	55.9	65.6	0.391
R	30	11	
44.1		34.4	
S	64	31	
Amikacin	94.1	96.9	1

		R	4	1
			5.9	3.1
		S	55	27
Gentamycin	80.9			84.4 0.785
		R	13	5
			19.1	15.6

ESBL

S :sensitive,**R** :resistant

1.5. Sensitivity according to the presence of underlying malformative uropathy:

We divided the patients into two groups: one with known underlying uropathic malformations (n=79) and one without (n=21). We found a statistically significant difference with several antibiotics between the 2 groups, but no difference for ESBL strains (Table VI).

Table VI. Antibiotic sensitivity according to the presence or absence of underlying malformative uropathy

		Absence d'uropathie malformative	Uropathie malformative sous-jacente	p
		n / %	n / %	
Amoxicilline-acide clavulanique	S	17 / 81	44 / 55.7	0.044
	R	4 / 19	35 / 44.3	
Cefuroxime	S	18 / 85.7	40 / 50.6	0.005
	R	3 / 14.3	39 / 49.4	
Cefixime	S	18 / 85.7	41 / 51.9	0.006
	R	3 / 14.3	38 / 48.1	
Cefotaxime	S	18 / 85.7	20 / 62.5	0.668
	R	3 / 14.3	12 / 37.5	
Ceftazidime	S	18 / 85.7	48 / 60.8	0.039
	R	3 / 14.3	31 / 39.2	
Imipenème	S	21 / 100	78 / 98.7	1
	R	0 / 0	1 / 1.3	
TPM-SMX	S	38 / 55.9	21 / 65.6	0.391
	R	30 / 44.1	11 / 34.4	
Amikacine	S	21 / 100	74 / 93.5	0.587
	R	0 / 0	5 / 6.3	
Gentamycine	S	20 / 95.2	62 / 78.5	0.11
	R	1 / 4.8	17 / 21.5	
BLSE	OUI	3 / 14.3	26 / 32.9	0.112
	NON	18 / 85.7	53 / 67.1	

S :sensible,**R** :résistant

1.6. Sensitivity according to previous antibiotic prescription :

We studied sensitivity in patients who had not received antibiotic therapy in the three months preceding the UTI (n=52) and those who had received antibiotic therapy during this period (n=48). This factor was associated with a statistically significant difference in resistance to several antibiotic families, and also with the presence of ESBL strains, with a p=0.004 (Table VII).

Table VII. Antibiotic susceptibility according to whether or not antibiotics were previously prescribed

		Pas d'antibiothérapie dans les 3 mois précédents	Antibiothérapie dans les 3 mois précédents	p
		n	n	
		%	%	
Amoxicilline-acide clavulanique	S	31	30	
		64.6	57.7	0.541
	R	17	22	
		35.4	42.3	
Cefuroxime	S	35	23	
		72.9	44.2	0.005
	R	13	29	
		27.1	55.8	
Cefixime	S	37	24	
		77.1	46.2	0.002
	R	11	28	
		22.9	53.8	
Cefotaxime	S	35	24	
		72.9	46.2	0.008
	R	13	28	
		27.1	53.8	
Ceftazidime	S	39	27	
		81.3	51.9	0.003
	R	9	25	
		18.8	48.1	
Imipenème	S	48	51	
		100	98.1	1
	R	0	1	
		0	1.9	
TPM-SMX	S	33	26	
		68.8	50	0.069
	R	15	26	
		31.3	50	
Amikacine	S	47	48	
		97.9	92.3	0.364
	R	1	4	
		2.1	7.7	
Gentamycine	S	43	39	
		89.6	75	0.071
	R	5	13	
		10.4	25	
BLSE	OUI	7	22	
		31.8	42.3	0.004
	NON	22	30	
		68.2	57.7	

S :sensible, R :résistant

1.7. **Sensitivity according to previous hospitalizations :**

We divided the patients into two groups: one that had been hospitalized in the months preceding the UTI (n=77) and one that had not been hospitalized prior to the infectious episode (n=23). We found a statistically significant difference for certain CIIIG molecules, but no difference for BLSE strains (Table VIII).

Table VIII. Antibiotic susceptibility according to the presence or absence of previous hospitalization

		Absence d'hospitalisation antérieure n %	Hospitalisation antérieure n %	p
Amoxicilline-acide clavulanique	S	16 69.6	45 58.4	0.466
	R	7 30.4	32 41.6	
Cefuroxime	S	18 78.3	40 51.9	0.031
	R	5 21.7	37 48.1	
Cefixime	S	19 82.6	42 54.5	0.016
	R	4 17.4	35 45.5	
Cefotaxime	S	18 78.3	41 53.2	0.052
	R	5 21.7	36 48.6	
Ceftazidime	S	19 82.6	47 61	0.078
	R	4 17.4	30 39	
Imipenème	S	23 100	76 98.7	1
	R	0 0	1 1.3	
TPM-SMX	S	18 78.3	41 53.2	0.052
	R	5 21.7	36 46.8	
Amikacine	S	23 100	72 93.5	0.587
	R	0 0	5 6.5	
Gentamycine	S	22 95.7	60 77.9	0.065
	R	1	17	
BLSE		4.3 3	22.1 26	0.068
	OUI	15	33.7	
	NON	20	51	
		85	66.3	

S :sensible,R :résistant

1.8. Sensitivity according to antibiotic prophylaxis :

We divided the patients into two groups: one on antibiotic prophylaxis (n=14) and one not on prophylaxis (n=86). No statistically significant difference was found between the 2 groups (Table IX).

Table IX. Antibiotic susceptibility according to whether or not antibiotic prophylaxis was taken

		Absence d'antibioprophylaxie	Antibioprophylaxie	p
		n %	n %	
Amoxicilline-acide clavulanique	S	52 60.5	9 64.3	1
	R	34 39.5	5 35.7	
Cefuroxime	S	49 57	9 64.3	0.772
	R	37 43	5 35.7	
Cefixime	S	52 60.5	9 64.3	1
	R	34 39.5	5 35.7	
Cefotaxime	S	50 58.1	9 64.3	0.774
	R	36 41.9	5 35.7	
Ceftazidime	S	56 65.1	10 71.4	0.767
	R	30 34.9	4 28.6	
Imipenème	S	85 98.8	14 100	1
	R	1 1.2	0 0	
TPM-SMX	S	52 60.5	7 50	0.561
	R	34 39.5	7 50	
Amikacine	S	81 94.2	31 96.9	1
	R	5	1	
Gentamycine	S	5.8 69 80.2	3.1 13 92.9	0.455
	R	17 19.8	1 7.1	
BLSE	OUI	25 29	4 28.5	1
	NON	61 71	10 71.5	

S :sensible,R :résistant

1.9. **Sensitivity according to the practice of intermittent catheterization or the presence of an indwelling catheter :**

We divided the patients into 2 groups: a first group whose patients did not use intermittent catheterization and had no indwelling bladder catheter (n=85); and a second group whose patients did use intermittent catheterization or had an indwelling bladder catheter (n=15).We found no statistically significant difference between these two groups for the different antibiotics tested.

2. Multi-variety study :

2.1. **Study of risk factors associated with the presence of an ESBL strain:**

The multivariate study looked for which of the variables tested and considered as risk factors for antibiotic resistance were associated with the presence of an ESBL strain (Table X):

Table X. Multivariate analysis of factors associated with the presence of an
ESBL strain

VariablesBSEB strain

independent

	Bivariate analysis ORb [95% CI] p	Multi-variate analysis ORa [95% CI] p
Gender	0.993	
Male Female	Ref. 1.004 [0.412-2.445]	
Age groups (months)	0.332	0.33
0-1 month	Ref.	Ref.
1-24 months	0.524[0.092-2.969]	1.3[0.15-11]
24-72 months	0.733[0.108-4.992]	1.7[0.15-19]
>72 months	1.33[0.225-7.89]	3.43[0.33-35]
Previous hospitalization	0.066	0.055
No	Ref.	Ref.
Yes	3.4 [0.92-12.49]	2[0.09-42]
Fever	0.73	
NO	Ref.	

YES	0.853[0.341-2.132]	
Intermittent surveys	0.31	
NO	Ref.	
YES	0.556[0.178-1.737]	
Malformative uropathy	0.11	0.09
NO	Ref.	Ref.
YES	2.94 [0.8-10.9]	1.03[0.12-8.7]
Recurrence of UTIs	0.084	0.07
NO	Ref.	Ref.
YES	3.16[0.858-11.68]	1.21[0.07-21]
Antibiotic prophylaxis	0.97	
NO	Ref.	
YES	0.976[0.28-3.4]	
Antibiotic therapy within 3	0.003	0.002
previous months NO	Ref.	Ref.
YES	4.29[1.625-11.355]	3.34[1.1-10.18]

A total of five factors were introduced into the initial multivariate analysis model:

- Previous hospitalization: the presence of a ESBL strain was more frequent in patients who had been hospitalized, taking patients who had not previously been hospitalized as the reference category (ORb =3.4; IC95%= [0.92-12.49]).

-Presence of underlying malformative uropathy:the presence of a BLSE strain was more frequent in patients with malformative uropathy taking patients without malformative uropathy as the reference category (ORb=2.94; IC95%= [0.8-10.9]).

- Recurrence of UTIs: the presence of a ESBL strain was more frequent in patients with previous infectious episodes, taking patients without UTI episodes as the reference category (ORb =3.16; IC95%= [0.858- 11.68]).

- Antibiotic treatment in the previous 3 months: the presence of a ESBL strain was more frequent in patients who had received antibiotic treatment in the previous 3 months, taking patients who had not received antibiotics in the previous 3 months as the reference category (ORb =4.29; IC95%= [1.625-

11.355]).

-The age group variable was considered as a forced variable (p=0.332) given its presence as a risk factor associated with antibiotic resistance in several studies. The reference category was 0-1 months, but the multivariate study found no statistical impact of the variable studied on the presence of ESBL strains.

The Wald-type top-down method concluded that the most parsimonious model contained only the variable prior antibiotic therapy in the preceding 3 months, with an OR of 3.34 and a p =0.002.

2.2. Validity of the binary logistic regression models used :

The logistic regression models were validated using several parameters: the pseudo R- two (Cox and Snell, Nagelkerke adjusted), the Hosmer-Lemeshow test and data from the classification table. Thus, for the model containing 5 variables in multivariate analysis, Nagelkerke's pseudo R-two was 18.7%. The model containing 5 variables shows an overall percentage of classification of observations of 70%.The Hosmer-Lemeshow test for the step containing 5 variables was non-significant with a value of p=0.47.

DISCUSSION

In our retrospective study of 100 episodes of UTI, the final logistic regression model retained a single independent risk factor for the occurrence of UTI with an ESBL-producing strain of enterobacteria, namely antibiotic use during the preceding 3 months.The results also enabled us to determine the bacterial ecosystem and emerging resistances within our department. The results showed that bacteria remained sensitive to the following molecules: nitrofurantoin, ciprofloxacin, gentamicin and amikacin, but showed increased resistance to amoxicillin-clavulanic acid, first-, second- and third-generation cephalosporins and TPM-SMX, making it necessary to rationalize the prescription of these antibiotics. Malformative uropathies were also a risk factor for resistance to amoxicillin-clavulanic acid and cephalosporins. We also found no carbapenase-secreting strains, and this therapeutic class remains a possible treatment option for ESBL strains. These bacteriological data are essential for establishing an empirical therapeutic strategy according to our own bacteriological map. To the best of our knowledge, our study was the first Tunisian study to examine risk factors for ESBL UTIs in paediatric settings. One of the main limitations of this study was its retrospective design, but thanks to the completeness of the records, particularly the computerized medical record, we had no missing data. In addition, certain potential confounding factors could not be studied, as reflected by a low Nagelkerke pseudo R- two of around 18.7%. In what follows, we begin with an overview of binary logistic regression modelling and then compare our results with those of the literature.

I. LOGISTIC REGRESSION :

1. The value of logistic regression in the analysis of data relating to medical practices :

When working with medical data, epidemiologists often have to describe an event or phenomenon that is itself influenced by the occurrence of other events or phenomena, known as exposure factors. The type of multivariate analysis chosen depends on the dependent variable. Logistic regression is used when the dependent variable is discrete, usually dichotomous. The variables On the other hand, independent variables can be qualitative or quantitative. The dependent variable is usually the occurrence or non-occurrence of an event, and the independent variables are those likely to influence the occurrence of this event, i.e. variables measuring exposure to a risk or protective factor, or variables representing a confounding factor (11).

To perform a regression is to attempt to reduce the data of a complex phenomenon to a simplifying mathematical law. The logistic function has a number of mathematical characteristics that explain its use in an epidemiological data analysis model: it varies from 0 to 1, like the probability of an event occurring; its graphical representation, in the form of a sigmoid, corresponds fairly closely to the model of the relationship between the occurrence of a disease and an exposure factor; finally, it enables odds ratios to be calculated. These measure the association of a given factor with the occurrence of an event. The odds ratio varies between zero and infinity. In the absence of association, it tends towards 1, and conversely when the variables are strongly linked, it tends towards zero or infinity. Although adaptations can be made to apply it to certain special cases, the logistic regression model requires, in principle, certain conditions: independence of the various observations from each other, normality of the distribution of the continuous variables included in the model, and linearity of the continuous independent variables in the logit.

2. Building the logistic model :

The practical implementation of a logistic regression model involves several steps (12,13):

2.1. Review of the literature and determination of variables :

The quality of a logistic regression depends above all on the choice of explanatory variables to be included in the model. This choice is based on clinical relevance and knowledge of known or suspected confounding factors. For this reason, a thorough literature search is a prerequisite (14).

2.2. Bivariate analysis :

We then proceed to analyze the links between each of the explanatory variables and the dependent variable, and between the explanatory variables themselves. The objectives of this step are: to generate crude ORs (odds ratios) and thus assess the strength of the relationship between the dependent variable and the explanatory variable. of the association between the independent variables and the dependent variable, assess the degree of collinearity between two explanatory variables, search for possible confounding factors and select the variables to be introduced into the logistic model. Thus, in bivariate analysis (two variables present in the study), several cases arise:

- The dependent variable is continuous, the independent variable is dichotomous (two-category categorical). If there is a match, we use the paired t-test if the distribution is normal, or the Wilcoxon test if the variable does not have a normal distribution. If there is no match, use the independent sample t-test if the distribution is normal, or the Mann-Whitney test if the distribution is abnormal.

-The independent variable is continuous, the dependent variable is categorical with more than two categories: we use the ANOVA test if the distribution is normal or the Kruskal-Wallis test if the distribution is abnormal.

-The independent and dependent variables are dichotomous. If there is a match, we use Mac Nemar's Chi-square test; if there is no match, we use Pearson's Chi-square test.

-If the independent variable and the dependent variable are categorical in more than two categories, we use the Pearson Chi-square test. If the two dependent variables are categorical, the Pearson Chi-square test is used.

-If the independent and dependent variables are continuous, we use Pearson's correlation if the distribution is normal, or Spearman's correlation if the distribution is abnormal; if the independent and dependent variables are continuous, we use simple linear regression.

-The independent variable is dichotomous and the dependent variable is a time variable, using the Logrank test.

The sample size required for both bivariate and multivariate analysis depends on the effect you are trying to demonstrate. The sample must be larger to demonstrate a moderate difference than to show a strong association between an independent variable and the outcome. Software is available to determine the number of patients required. In our work, we we calculated the number of subjects required to obtain 5% accuracy for UTI prevalence estimates in children, based on the following formula: $n = (1.96)2 * P0 * (1-P0) \setminus i2$

n= Number of subjects required

P0= prevalence of UTIs in children. i= 0.05

In order to guarantee the stability of the multivariate model, a rule often used is that for each variable to be included in the model, between 5 and 10 cases of the least frequent modality of the explained variable are required. In our study, the dependent variable studied was the presence of ESBL strains, with the least represented modality accounting for a total of 29 patients. We thus introduced 5 variables into the regression model. The choice of variables to be introduced into the logistic model is based on a combination of scientific knowledge of the problem, the use of statistical methods, experience and common sense. The aim is to arrive at the best model for the question at hand, taking into account scientifically important variables, controlling confounding phenomena and ensuring the stability of the results so that they can be extrapolated. A balance must be struck between, on the one hand, too many factors being taken into account, which could lead to a loss of power, over-fitting or the generation of unstable, less interpretable results, and on the other hand, too few factors being taken into account, leading to possible residual confounding and a poorer fit of the model. Thus, the independent variables to be included in the logistic model are the risk factors of interest and the variables that potentially play a confounding role between the variables of interest and the dependent variable, as summarized in the theoretical model. Redundant variables, variables with more than 3% missing data and variables that are an integral part of the causal scheme are excluded. Three types of variables are included in the initial model: those for which the association with the dependent variable in the bivariate analysis is sufficiently strong, but not so strict as to omit possible confounding factors (14) (p ≤ 0.1 or even 0.2, and not 0.05, the threshold usually used); those of proven clinical interest outside any association criteria, known as forced variables; and the confounding variables described in the literature or identified in the bivariate analysis.

2.3. Initial logistic model :

This step consists in building the regression model using :
-All variables with a significance level of less than 0.20 (i.e. with a p-value < 0.20) in the univariate analysis. This threshold of 0.20, and not 0.05 as usually used in statistics, allows us to take into account variables that could be possible confounding or interaction factors. Of course, such a threshold may seem arbitrary and may vary according to the habits of different teams (it is

sometimes 0.25, sometimes 0.30). Variables known to be associated with disease will also be included in the analysis, even if uni-variate analysis did not result in a p<0.20 value. These are known as "forced" variables.

2.4. Final model :

There are several possible strategies for arriving at a final model, which should carry the maximum amount of information while having a limited number of variables to facilitate interpretation: the most commonly used are the so-called "step-by-step descending" or "step-by-step ascending" procedures. In our study, the occurrence of anti-bio-resistance such as the presence of a ESBL strain is the dependent variable, and the independent variables are those that constitute potential risk factors for the occurrence of an antibiotic- or ESBL-resistant UTI, and were as follows:age, gender, previous hospitalization, fever lasting more than 48 hours, intermittent catheterization or indwelling bladder catheter, underlying malformative uropathy, recurrence of UTI, prior antibiotic prophylaxis and antibiotic therapy within the previous 3 months.

II. EPIDEMIOLOGICAL PROFILEOF URINARY TRACT INFECTIONSIN CHILDREN:

1. Age and gender

Our study showed a predominance of UTIs in infants, a predominance of boys in this age group, and a predominance of girls in children over two years of age. The age and sex distribution of children in our study is therefore in line with the literature (15). Studies carried out in Morocco in 2019 also showed a clear overall predominance of UTIs in boys before the age of three and in girls from the age of 3 (2), and that this predominance is even more marked between the ages of 6 and 16, with 2% in girls versus 0.1 % in boys (16,17). Similarly, in

Turkey, isolates were found in 84.3% of boys in patients under 2 years of age, and in 66.8% of girls in children over 2 years of age (7). In newborns and small infants, the predominance of males in UTIs is due to the high incidence of malformative uropathy and RVU in this age group. In pre-school age, girls are more affected than boys, due to anatomical peculiarities and poor hygiene (18). Other studies in Turkey have found concordant results, and this difference could be associated with the lack of circumcision among young boys, as neonatal circumcision is not widespread in Turkey (19-21), with a lower incidence of UTIs among circumcised boys (22).

2. Overall bacteriological profile :

The most common germs in our study were, in order of frequency:Esherichia coli(66%) followed by Klebsiella pneumoniae (14%) and Pseudomonas aeruginosa (7 In Morocco, too, Escherichia coli dominated the epidemiological profile (39%), followed by Klebsiella pneumoniae (21%) and Enterococcus spp (12%), with the remainder shared between yeasts, Pseudomonas aeruginosa and other Enterobacteriaceae (6).Enterobacteriaceae dominate the bacteriological profile of UTIs, with Escherichia coli coming out on top, as also reported in the Moroccan study and in several international studies (2,6,23,24). Colonization of the perineum by enterobacteria of digestive origin, the ascending pathophysiology of UTI and specific bacterial uropathogenic factors such as adhesins explain this predominance, particularly for Escherichia coli (25). The study of germs by age group in our study showed that Esherichia coli was always the main etiological agent in the different age groups, followed by Klebsiella pneumoniae in infants and then Pseudomonas aeruginosa in older children, which is consistent with other studies (5).Three bacteria dominated the profile of UTI in newborns in Morocco: Klebsiella pneumoniae (29.9%), Escherichia coli (24.7%) and Enterococcus (23.4%). As age increased, Escherichia coli dominated the bacteriological profile (35% of cases in infants,

47% in children and 48% in older children) (p < 0.001). In the Turkish study, the majority of Esherichia coli were found in girls (79.6% vs. 55% in boys). Other species were more common in boys: Proteus , Klebsiella, Enterobacter, Enterococcus and Pseudomonas, with a statistically significant difference from girls for all these germs except Enterobacter (7).

3. Global antibiotic resistance :

Studies of the antibiotic sensitivity of strains responsible for UTI in children have shown very high rates of resistance to the antibiotics tested. These resistances have also been reported in various national, Maghrebian and European studies(6,22,26-28). The increase in resistance among our patients can be explained by the use of most of these antibiotics, in particular ampicillin, amoxicillin-clavulanic acid and cephalosporins, to treat other infections, notably respiratory and ENT, and as first-line probabilistic treatment for UTI (6,8).We studied the resistance of our ecology to the main antibiotics used in our current practice.

3.1. Resistance to amoxicillin/clavulanic acid :

In our study, resistance to this molecule was 39%. A study in Turkey revealed that overall resistance of microorganisms to amoxicillin-clavulanic acid was 47.6% (7). Amoxicillin-clavulanic acid is widely used for respiratory tract infections and otitis media in children, which explains this resistance. Two other studies indicated that the average sensitivity of all isolates was 19%, demonstrating that these antibiotics can no longer be used for the empirical treatment of UTIs in children in these regions (7,20,29).

3.2. TPM-SMX resistance :

TPM-SMX has been the most common first-line treatment for UTIs worldwide, as demonstrated by 3 studies in 15 different countries (30).In our study, resistance to this molecule was 41%. Al-Mugeiren et al in Saudi Arabia reported resistance of 67% in 596 isolates (30).In Turkey resistance to TPM-SMX increased from 2009 to 2014 (40.6% and 52.5%)(7).Other studies in Turkey reported resistance to TPM-SMX between 50% and 75.4% (20). Also in Morocco resistance to TPM-SMX in enterobacteria of all species affected one strain in 2 (53%).

3.3. Furantoin resistance :

In our study, resistance to this molecule was low at 9%. Our bacteriological profile therefore still allows effective first-line use of this molecule. Resistance to nitrofurantoin, an antibiotic used almost exclusively for UTIs, was low worldwide, supporting its continued efficacy as a first-line treatment for uncomplicated infections (30). On the other hand, a study in Turkey revealed an overall resistance of microorganisms to nitrofurantoin of 27.1%. Resistance rates of Esherichia coli, Proteus and Klebsiella to nitrofurantoin from 2009 to 2014 were 5.3-15.2%, 67.7-77.7% and 33.6-54.5%, respectively, and the use of this single antibiotic as empirical therapy for UTIs in Turkey has therefore been discontinued (7).

3.4. Resistance to cephalosporins :

Our study showed a resistance rate of 48% to first-generation cephalosporins and 42% to second-generation cephalosporins. Resistance to CIIIGs was also significant, with 39% resistance to cefixime, forty-one percent to cefotaxime and 34% to ceftazidime. The study by Ron Eremenko et al showed the lowest rate with first- and second-generation cephalosporins at 9.9% (5). Sheikh et al showed similar rates to Israel for resistance to first- and second-generation cephalosporins with Escherichia coli infections, but not with other germs, which is in line with another study carried out in Israel (5). In a study carried out in Iran, Esherichia coli and Klebsiella were the least resistant to cefuroxime (31). Studies carried out in Turkey showed that the rate of resistance of Escherichia coli to ceftriaxone fell from 21.1% in 2009 to 5.9% in 2014(5). Chen et al reported that the sensitivity rate of Escherichia coli to ceftriaxone was 85%(32). Esherichia coli resistance to cefuroxime was 24.1% in Turkey in 2014. (7). In Morocco, resistance to CIIIG in enterobacteria of all species was observed in 46% of isolates (2). This study concurs with other international studies on the worrying rates of resistance to CIIIG (2,8,33,34). The high level of resistance of enterobacteria to CIIIG found in our study and reported by various studies is the consequence of the selection pressure due to the massive prescription and often abusive use of CIIIG in both hospital and community settings, as well as the cross-transmission of acquired plasmid resistance (6).

3.5. Aminoglycoside resistance :

In our study, good antibiotic activity was recorded with aminoglycosides, gentamycin resistance was low at 18%, and the best antibiotic activity was recorded with amikacin, with only 9% of resistant strains. In another study, aminoglycosides maintained good activity, mainly amikacin and to a lesser extent gentamicin (6). Here too, our study and the latter are in line with international studies (2,35,35,36), making these molecules a good therapeutic alternative both as monotherapy and in combination.

3.6. Resistance to fluoroquinolones

Fluoroquinolone resistance in our series was 17% for ciprofloxacin and 18% for ofloxacin. Fluoroquinolones, which have very interesting anti-bacterial activity, should obviously be avoided in children until the end of the growth period, due to their joint toxicity, except in cases of resistance to other antibiotics, where their use remains possible in older children (6).

3.7. Carbapenem resistance :

In our study, ten percent of enterobacterial strains were resistant to ertapenem and only 1% to imipenem. The global prevalence of these strains varies from study to study, but spares virtually no country (34,37).In Morocco the rates of imipenem-resistant Klebsiella and Proteus tended to increase from 2009 to 2014. The increase in carbapenem consumption has led to the emergence of a new resistance mechanism: carbapenemases (33,37,38).this should alert us to the ease of use of carbapenems and their current interest in the treatment strategy (7).

3.8. ESBL strains :

In our study, the frequency of ESBL strains was 29%. In the study carried out in Morocco in 2019, 13% of enterobacteria strains were ESBL (6). This frequency is significantly higher than that reported at Moulay-Ismail Hospital in Meknes between 2006-2008 (9%) and at Caen University Hospital in France in 2014 (4.5%). In In our study, only the use of antibiotics during the previous 3 months was associated with the presence of a ESBL strain. This same factor was found in other studies, which also showed that underlying neurological disease, recent hospitalization and community care were the main risk factors for ESBL UTIs in pediatrics (39,40). In other studies, recurrent UTIs were the risk factor significantly associated with ESBL germs (41,42). Enterobacteriaceae ESBL have spread throughout the world, and beyond the hospital setting. Indeed, these strains are now widespread not only among community patients, but also in the environment. This is a consequence of the extensive antibiotic therapy used in agriculture and veterinary medicine, and explains why they are now found on animal farms, in pets and in rivers (33). Moreover, ESBL production has an impact on resistance to other antibiotics. High rates of resistance in ESBL-producing strains have been found in comparison with CIIIG-susceptible strains (43,44). Furthermore, 50%, 30% and 60% of ESBL-producing strains are resistant to fluoroquinolones, aminoglycosides and TMP-SMX respectively (2). Treatment of these multi-resistant strains is therefore restricted to carbapenems, colistin, fosfomycin, nitrofurantoin and tigecycline (45). Fosfomycin and nitrofurantoin can only be used in the treatment of lower UTIs. Colistin also remains effective, but carries a high risk of toxicity due to its very narrow therapeutic index. Tigecycline is contraindicated before the age of 8, and has no urinary diffusion (45). For these reasons, carbapenems have always been the treatment of suspected or documented ESBL-producing enterobacterial infections. Today, with the emergence of carbapenemases, the use of carbapenems is limited.

3.9. BMR strains :

Of the ESBL germs isolated in our study, 96.5% were MDR; in fact, 28% of the strains isolated in UTI in children in our study were MDR; the same finding was found in the study carried out at the Yopougon University Hospital between 2014-2015, with a rate of 29.7% (46). Among these isolated BMR, enterobacteriaceae occupied first place, and Escherichia coli was the species most affected by multiresistance, as also reported in Marrakech by Moutachakkir el al (47). The problem of bacterial resistance in pediatric UTI is therefore mainly a question of Enterobacteriaceae, with the increase in resistance to CIIIG and the emergence of strains with reduced sensitivity to carbapenems. The major risk is currently posed by ESBL strains and carbapenemase-secreting strains, which can combine to generate pan-resistance (6).

III. FACTORS OF RISK ASSOCIATED A THE RESISTANCE TO ANTIBIOTICS :

1. Age :

Our study showed higher resistance in newborns, with a statistically significant difference according to age with amoxicillin-clavulanic acid and gentamycin, but no difference for ESBL strains in univariate analysis. In the initial model, the p was equal to 0.332, so this variable was considered a forced variable, but in multi-variate analysis we found no statistical impact of this variable on the presence of ESBL strains.A meta-analysis carried out in 2016 revealed higher resistance in children aged 0 to 5 in developing countries than in developed countries. This meta-analysis found Escherishia coli resistance in children aged 0-5 higher for ampicillin and ceftazidime, and lower for amoxicillin-clavulanic acid, TMP-SMX and nitrofurantoin in developed countries. In developing countries, resistance was higher for all antibiotics in children aged 0 to 5 than in other age groups (30).These resistance levels are higher in younger children, due to higher antibiotic consumption in this age group (48). A study carried out in France showed that children under 7 years of age consume three times more antibiotics than older populations (49).Our results are in line with the group of developing countries, since the majority of antibiotics, including those used to treat UTIs, are obtained without a doctor's prescription, unlike in developed countries, where antibiotics are only available on prescription.

2.Recurrence of urinary tract infections:

In our study, we found no statistically significant difference between patients with repeated UTIs in univariate analysis for the different antibiotics and for ESBL strains.Recurrent UTI was a risk factor for the occurrence of ESBL strains introduced in the initial logistic regression model (ORb=3.16; CI [0.858-11.68], p= 0.084), but was not retained in the final model. The study by Ron

Eremenko et al showed a statistically significant difference with amoxicillin-clavulanic acid between the two groups; first UTI group and recurrent UTI group; but not with first- and second-generation cephalosporins. Other studies have shown that the factor associated with anti-bio-resistance was not the number of infectious episodes, but the presence of underlying malformative uropathy at the origin of these recurrent UTIs; in particular, the presence of a UTI was a risk factor for the appearance of resistant germs, notably Escherichia coli ESBL (50,51).

3. Malformative uropathy:

In our study, univariate analysis showed that the presence of malformative uropathy was associated with antibiotic resistance to amoxicillin-clavulanic acid (p=0.044), cefuroxime (p=0.005), cefixime (p=0.006) and ceftazidime (p=0.039). In multivariate analysis, this variable was included in the initial logistic regression model (ORb=2.94; CI [0.8-10.9], p= 0.11), but was not retained in the final model as an independent risk factor for antibiotic resistance.

Other studies have also investigated the association of uropathy with antibiotic resistance, and have highlighted resistance to a number of antibiotics, notably ceftriaxone and cefixime; this is in line with our results, with a statistically significant difference for resistance to CIIIG, notably cefixime (52).

4. Previous hospitalization :

In our study, univariate analysis showed that prior hospitalization was associated with antibiotic resistance with cefuroxime (p=0.031) and cefixime (p=0.006). In multivariate analysis, prior hospitalization was included in the initial logistic regression model (ORb=3.4; CI [0.92-12.49], p= 0.066), but was not retained in the final model as an independent risk factor for antibiotic resistance. Hospitalization is likely to generate antibiotic resistance through the colonization of children by hospital-acquired germs, particularly ESBL strains. Indeed, ESBL strains of enterobacteria have emerged over the last 25 years, first causing nosocomial epidemics and then spreading throughout the world, creating a pandemic situation (40). Hospitalization may also be responsible for the acquisition of antibiotic resistance, of course, if antibiotics are prescribed during hospitalization.

5. Previous antibiotic prescriptions :

Our study showed a statistically significant difference between patients who had or had not received antibiotics in the 3 months prior to UTI for second- and third-generation cephalosporins. Antibiotic use was also associated with the presence of ESBL strains in univariate analysis (p=0.003) and in multivariate analysis. Ron Eremenko et al found no statistically significant difference between patients who had or had not received antibiotics in the 2 years prior to UTI (5) and Brosh Nissimov et al between patients who had or had not received antibiotics in the 6 months prior to UTI (53), although the latter demonstrated that prescribing fluoroquinoles or cephalosporins during this period could lead to antibiotic resistance. Other studies have shown that patients who have been treated in the last six months can develop resistance to cephalosporins or amoxicillin (51). A meta-analysis of Esherichia coli UTIs showed a difference in resistance to these bacteria in cases of prior antibiotic prescription, particularly with regard to TMP-SMX and ciprofloxacin (30). Topaloglu et al showed that children who had received antibiotics in the 3 months preceding the infectious episode developed resistance to CIIIG (54). Allen et al demonstrated that antibiotic use in the 6 months preceding the infectious episode generated resistance to TMP-SMX.(55). The 2016 meta-analysis on E coli UTIs demonstrated that prescribing antibiotics to children in primary care contributes significantly to bacterial resistance, which can persist for up to six months after prescription (30). This meta-analysis showed that these antibiotics are used differently in different countries, which explains the difference in molecules to which resistance has emerged. Furthermore, none of the studies included in this meta-analysis reported the doses of antibiotics and it was therefore impossible to assess the effects of the dose-effect relationship.

CONCLUSIONS

Bacteriological and epidemiological data play a decisive role in the management of UTIs in children. The prescription of empirical antibiotics takes into account the susceptibility of the target organisms to antibiotics, and so knowledge of the level of resistance is essential. A resistance rate of 20% has been considered acceptable for first-line probabilistic antibiotic therapy (5). Our study looked at resistance rates to antibiotics, particularly those prescribed as first-line empirical treatment for UTIs in children.In this study, we carried out a cross-sectional etiological study on a series of children admitted for UTI. All urine samples from children hospitalized in the pediatric nephrology department from January to September 2020 were examined in the bacteriology department of Charles Nicolle Hospital. We included all children admitted for suspected UTI to the pediatric nephrology department and whose infection was confirmed by a positive culture of the ECBU. We collected data relating to the interview, clinical and paraclinical examinations carried out during hospitalization. The analytical study used appropriate tests: Pearson's Chi2 test and, in the event of invalidity, Fisher's test and logistic regression. Our aim was to identify the risk factors associated with the occurrence of ESBL-producing UTI in children. A total of 100 bacteriologically confirmed episodes of UTI were included in the study. The 100 episodes involved 100 patients. There were 38 boys and 62 girls. The sex ratio was 0.6. The average age of all patients was 59.7 months, with extremes ranging from 3 days to 17 years. In newborns and infants, UTIs mainly affected boys, whereas in children and older children, females were most affected; with a significant gender distribution ($p < 0.001$). Escherichia coli dominated the epidemiological profile (66%), followed by Klebsiella pneumoniae (14%) and Pseudomonas aeruginosa (7%).two bacteria dominated the UTI profile in newborns: Escherichia coli (66%) and Klebsiella pneumoniae (14%). In other age groups, Escherichia coli dominated the bacteriological profile, followed by Klebsiella pneumoniae in infants and Pseudomonas in children over 2 years of age. In our study, the most isolated germ was Escherichia coli in both girls and boys.Overall antibiotic susceptibility across all germs showed 39% resistance t o amoxicillin/clavulanic acid; forty-eight percent to first-generation cephalosporins, forty-two percent to second-generation cephalosporins, thirty-nine percent to cefixime, forty-one percent to cefotaxime, thirty-four percent to ceftazidime and 41% to TPM- SMX. Nitrofurantoin, fluoroquinolones and aminoglycosides were the most active molecules, with resistance rates of 9%, 17%, 18% and 18% respectively. 5% respectively for nitrofurantoin, ciprofloxacin, gentamicin and amikacin. In univariate analysis, we found a statistically significant difference in sensitivity to amxicillin/clavulanic acid across age groups and gender.The presence of malformative uropathy was associated with resistance to amoxicillin-clavulanic acid (p=0.044), cefuroxime (p= 0.005), cefixime (p= 0.006) and ceftazidime (p=0.039).Analysis of antibiotic sensitivity according to whether or not antibiotics had been prescribed in the previous 3 months showed a statistically significant difference with cefuroxime (p= 0.005), cefixime (p= 0.002) and ceftazidime (p= 0.008). Previous hospitalization, intermittent catheterization or the presence of an indwelling bladder catheter were not associated with antibiotic resistance.No factor studied was associated with the presence of a ESBL strain in univariate analysis. Five factors associated with the presence of an ESBL strain were introduced into the initial model of the multivariate analysis:

- Previous hospitalization: the presence of a ESBL strain was more frequent in patients who had been hospitalized previously (ORb=3.4; IC95%= [0.92-12.49]).

-Presence of underlying malformative uropathy:the presence of a BLSE strain was more frequent in patients with malformative uropathy (ORb =2.94, IC95%= [0.8-10.9]).

- Recurrence of UTIs: the presence of a ESBL strain was more frequent in patients with previous infectious episodes (ORb =3.16; IC95%= [0.858- 11.68]).

- Antibiotics taken in the previous 3 months: the presence of an ESBL strain was more frequent in patients who had received antibiotic treatment in the previous 3 months (ORb=4.29; IC95%= [1.625-11.355]).

- Age was considered a forced variable given its presence as a risk factor associated with antibiotic resistance in several studies, but the multivariate study found no statistical impact on the presence of ESBL strains.

The Wald-type top-down method concluded with the most parsimonious model containing only the variable prior antibiotic therapy in the previous 3 months with an ORa at 3.34, a 95% CI ranging from 1.1 to 10.18, and a p =0.002.

Thus, for the model containing 5 variables in multivariate analysis, Nagelkerke's pseudo R-two was 18.7%. The Hosmer-Lemeshow test for the 5-variable step was insignificant, with a p=0.63 value. Our results confirm the evolving and worrying nature of antibiotic resistance in uropathogenic germs, detailing the overall high level of resistance to some of the most commonly prescribed antibiotics in children, demonstrating the ineffectiveness of these molecules as first-line treatment for UTI.In fact, the Infectious Diseases Society of America, in collaboration with the European Society for Microbiology and Infectious Diseases, specifies that antibiotics should only be chosen for empirical first-line treatment of UTI if the local prevalence of resistance is less than 20% (4). In order to avoid the selection of more resistant strains, continuous monitoring of resistance, rational antibiotic prescription by primary care physicians and hygiene measures for patients infected with or carrying BMR are essential (2).It is essential to improve the conditions under which we diagnose UTIs, in order to avoid unnecessary treatment. Furthermore, antibiotic sparing in cases of urinary tract colonization is a genuine means of combating antibiotic resistance (6).In cases of UTI, we must apply the current recommendations for the management of UTIs, taking into account the particularities of our local bacterial ecology and the data on antibiotic resistance generated by our study. The choice of appropriate antibiotic therapy should follow a guideline based on the specific parameters of each patient.It is also important to avoid the use of carbapenems in UTIs with ESBL-producing strains, in order to avoid the emergence of carbapenemase-secreting strains, and to consider the possibility of monotherapy with an aminoglycoside or a combination of amoxicillin and clavulanic acid when the minimum inhibitory concentration is active and the child's clinical condition permits (6). Other studies suggest the possibility of combining cefixime with amoxicillin/clavulanic acid, after verifying the in vitro synergy of amoxicillin/clavulanic acid and cefixime in a laboratory with mastery of the technique, with a MIC of the combination < 1 mg/L (52). Lastly, prospective epidemiological studies requiring ongoing cooperation between clinicians and microbiologists are essential, with a dual objective: therapeutic, to guide treatment strategy, and prophylactic, to identify and remedy antibiotic resistance factors.

REFERENCES

1. Ricco R. Pratique de la régression logistique [Online]. Université Lumière Lyon. [cited 2011 June]. Available from URL: https://eric.univ-lyon2.fr/~ricco/cours/cours/pratique_ regression_logistique.pdf.

2. Maleb A, Lahrache K, Lamrabat S, Rifai S, Rahmani N, Bensalah M, et al. Infantile urinary tract infections at the Mohammed VI University Hospital in Oujda . J Pediatrie Puériculture.2019;32(6):322-9.

3. Frédéric J,Elvire MK,Audrey M,JD C. Les difficultés d'interprétation de l'examen cytobactériologique des urines. Encycl Med Chir (Elsevier Masson, Paris), Archives de pédiatrie, Vol 16 - N° 7, 2009, 7p.

4. Iacobelli S, Bonsante F. Infections urinaires en pédiatrie Encycl Med Chir (Elsevier Masson, Paris), Revue francophone des laboratoires, 406, 2008, 9p.

5. Eremenko R, Barmatz S, Lumelsky N, Colodner R, Strauss M, Alkan Y. Urinary Tract Infection in Outpatient Children and Adolescents: Risk Analysis of Antimicrobial

Resistance. Isr Med Assoc J.2020;22(4):236-40.

6. Zahir H, Draiss G, Rada N, Abourrahouat A, Aitsab I, Sbihi M, et al. Microbial ecology and antibiotic susceptibility of bacteria isolated from urinary tract infections in children in Morocco. Rev Francoph Lab.2019;(511):65-70.

7. Erol B, Culpan M, Caskurlu H, Sari U, Cag Y, Vahaboglu H, et al. Changes in antimicrobial resistance and demographics of UTIs in pediatric patients in a single institution over a 6-year period. J Pediatr Urol.2018;14(2):176.e1-176.e5.

8. Cohen R, Raymond J, Faye A,Gillet Y,Grimprel E . Management of urinary tract infections in children. Recommendations of the Pediatric Infectious Pathology Group of the French Pediatric Society and the Société de pathologie

infectieuse de langue française. Encycl Med Chir (Elsevier Masson, Paris), Archives de pédiatrie, Vol 22 - N° 6, 2015, 7p.

9. Glissmeyer EW, Korgenski EK, Wilkes J, Schunk JE, Sheng X, Blaschke AJ, et al. Dipstick screening for urinary tract infection in febrile infants.Pediatrics.2014;133(5):1121-27.

10. Canis F.Référentiel en microbiologie médicale (REMIC).6ème edition.France: Société Française de Microbiologie SFM; 2018.

11. Aminot I, Damon MN. Logistic regression: interest in the analysis of data relating to medical practices.Revue médicale de l'assurance maladie. 2002; 137-43.

12. ES M, Naudet F. Understanding logistic regression. J Fr Ophthalmol. 2013;36(8):710-5.

13. Preux PM,Odermatt P ,Perna A,Marin B,Vergnenègre A· What is logistic regression? Encycl Med Chir (Elsevier Masson, Paris), Revue des maladies respiratoires, Vol 22 - N° 1, 2005, 4p.

14. Preux PM, Odermatt P, Perna A, Marin B, Vergnenègre A. Logistic regression. Rev Mal Respir.2005;22:159-62.

15. Bouskraoui M, AS I, Draiss G, Bourrouss M, Sbihi M. Epidemiology of urinary tract infection in children in Marrakech. Arch Pediatr Organe Off Soc Francaise Pediatr.2010;17 Suppl 4:177-8.

16. Lagree M, Bontemps S, Dessein R, Angoulvant F, Madhi F, Martinot A, et al. Extended- spectrum β-lactamase-producing Enterobacteriaceae, national study of antimicrobial treatment for pediatric urinary tract infection. Med Mal Infect. 2018;48(3):193-201.

17. Carole E. Investigation of a urinary tract infection in children. Encycl Med Chir (Elsevier Masson, Paris), Option bio, Vol 19 - N° 396, 2008, p19.

18. Iacobelli S, F. Bonsante F, JP G. Exploration d'une infection urinaire de l'enfant. Encycl Med Chir (Elsevier Masson, Paris), Archives de pédiatrie, Vol 16 - N° 7, 2009, 7p.

19. Beetz R, Westenfelder M. Antimicrobial therapy of urinary tract infections in children. Int J Antimicrob Agents.2011;38 Suppl:42-50.

20. Seyed RM ,Morteza S, Masoud SB, Masoud R,Mojtaba M.Bacterial Pathogens and Antimicrobial Resistance Patterns in Pediatric Urinary Tract Infections: A Four-Year Surveillance Study (2009-2012).Int J of Pediatrics.2014;1-6

21. Badhan R, Singh DV, Badhan LR, Kaur A. Evaluation of bacteriological profile and antibiotic sensitivity patterns in children with urinary tract infection: A prospective study.
from a tertiary care center. Indian J Urol. 2016;32(1):50-6.

22. Yolbaş I, Tekin R, Kelekci S, Tekin A, Okur MH, Ece A, et al. Community-acquired urinary tract infections in children: pathogens, antibiotic susceptibility and seasonal changes. Eur Rev Med Pharmacol.2013;17(7):971-6.

23. IIW RII, Ghanem ST, EH MW, Khafaja SA, Shaker RA, Hassan SA, et al. Epidemiology and characteristics of urinary tract infections in children and adolescents. Front Cell Infect Microbiol. 2015;5:45.

24. Wani KA, Ashraf M, Bhat JA, Parry NA, Shaheen L, Bhat SA. Paediatric Urinary Tract Infection: A Hospital Based Experience. J Clin Diagn Res JCDR. 2016;10(10):SC04-7.

25. Larabi K. Étude bactériologique et phénotypes de résistance des germes responsables d'infections urinaires dans un CHU de Tunis : à propos de 1930 cas. Encycl Med Chir (Elsevier Masson, Paris), Médecine et maladies infectieuses, Vol 33 - N° 7, 2003, 5p.

26. Parajuli NP, Maharjan P, Parajuli H, Joshi G, Paudel D, Sayami S, et al. High rates of multidrug resistance among uropathogenic Escherichia coli in children and analyses of ESBL producers from Nepal. Antimicrob Resist Infect Control. 2017;6:9.

27. Garraffo A, Marguet C, Checoury A, Boyer S, Gardrat A, Houivet E, et al. Urinary tract infections in hospital pediatrics: many previous antibiotic treatments and antibiotic resistance,

including fluoroquinolones. Med Mal Infect.2014;44(2):63-8.

28. Oli AN, Akabueze VB, Ezeudu CE, Eleje GU, Ejiofor OS, Ezebialu IU, et al. Bacteriology and Antibiogram of Urinary Tract Infection Among Female Patients in a Tertiary Health Facility in South Eastern Nigeria. Open Microbiol J.2017;11:292-300.

29. Çoban B, Ülkü N, Kaplan H, Topal B, Erdoğan H, Baskın E. Five-year assessment of causative agents and antibiotic resistances in urinary tract infections. Turk Arch Pediatr Pediatri Arş.2014;49(2):124-9.

30. Bryce A, Hay AD, Lane IF, Thornton HV, Wootton M, Costelloe C. Global prevalence of antibiotic resistance in paediatric urinary tract infections caused by Escherichia coli and association with routine use of antibiotics in primary care: systematic review and meta- analysis. BMJ.2016;352:i939.

31. Sweih NA, Jamal W, Rotimi VO. Spectrum and Antibiotic Resistance of Uropathogens Isolated from Hospital and Community Patients with Urinary Tract Infections in Two Large Hospitals in Kuwait. Med Princ Pract. 2005;14(6):401-7.

32. Chen PC, Chang LY, Lu CY, Shao PL, Tsai IJ, Tsau YK, et al. Drug susceptibility and treatment response of common urinary tract infection pathogens in children. J Microbiol Immunol Infect Wei Mian Yu Gan Ran Za Zhi.2014;47(6):478-83.

.033. Vodovar D,Marcadé G,Raskine L,Malissin I , Mégarbane B. Extended-spectrum beta-lactamase-producing Enterobacteriaceae. Encycl Med Chir (Elsevier Masson, Paris),La revue de médecine interne, Vol 34 - N° 11, 2013, 7p.

34. Duong HP, MH TT, Hoang DT, Janssen F, Lepage P, DM P, et al. Difficulties in managing of infections at children Arch Pédiatrie.2015;22(8):848-52.

35. Bouskraoui M, AS I, Draiss G, Bourrouss M, Sbihi M. Epidemiology of urinary tract infection in children in Marrakech. Arch Pédiatrie.2010;17:S177-8.

36. Arsalane L, Zouhair S, Lahlou Amine I, Louzi L, Bouskraoui M. Infant urinary tract infection (376 cases) in a Moroccan hospital (2009-2010) - etiological frequency and
prevalence of resistance. Pathol Biol.2012;60(6):90-1.

37. Durrmeyer X, Cohen R. Use of carbapenems in pediatrics. Arch Pediatrie.2010;17:163-70.

38. Legeay C, Hilliquin D, Brunet M, Zahar J-R. Extended-spectrum beta-lactamases, what's the risk in oncopediatrics? Rev Oncol Hématologie Pédiatrique. 2016;4(1):25-34.

39. Flammang A, Morello R, Vergnaud M, Brouard J, Eckart P. Study of the bacterial resistance profile in pediatric pyelonephritis in 2014. Arch Pédiatrie.2017;24(3):215-24.

40. Bonacorsi S, MK P, Desmarest M, Doit C. Extended-spectrum beta-lactamase-producing Enterobacteriaceae in pediatrics 2014 update. Arch Pediatrie.2014;21(5, Supplement 1):181-2.

41. Flokas ME, Detsis M, Alevizakos M, Mylonakis E. Prevalence of ESBL-producing Enterobacteriaceae in paediatric urinary tract infections: A systematic review and meta- analysis. J Infect.2016;73(6):547-57.

42. Topaloglu R, Er I, Dogan BG, Bilginer Y, Ozaltin F, Besbas N, et al. Risk factors in community-acquired urinary tract infections caused by ESBL-producing bacteria in children. Pediatr Nephrol Berl Ger.2010;25(5):919-25.

43. LA M. Chegri M,Kassmi H. Epidemiology and antibiotic resistance of enterobacteria isolated from urinary tract infections at the Moulay-Ismail military hospital in Meknes. Encycl Med Chir (Elsevier Masson, Paris), Antibiotics, Vol 11 - N° 2, 2009, 4p.

44. Gupta P, Mandal J, Krishnamurthy S, Barathi D, Pandit N. Profile of urinary tract infections in paediatric patients. Indian J Med Res.2015;141(4):473-7.

45. Basmaci R, Cohen R. What should the pediatrician know about extended-spectrum beta- lactamase-producing Escherichia coli? Perfect En Pediatrie.2018;1(1):62-7.

46. BC C,Zaba F,Meite S et al.Profil bactériologique des infections urinaires en pédiatrie:cas du CHU du Yopougan.J sci pharm biol. 2015;1:34-41.

47. Moutachakkir M,Chinbo M,Elkhoudri N, Soraa N. Antibiotic resistance in uropathogenic Enterobacteriaceae in the pediatric setting at Marrakech University Hospital. Encycl Med Chir (Elsevier Masson, Paris),Journal de pédiatrie et de puériculture, Vol 28 - N° 1, 2015, 7p.

48. Turnidge J, Christiansen K. Antibiotic use and resistance--proving the obvious. Lancet Lond Engl.2005;365(9459):548-9.

49. Sommet A. No significant decrease in antibiotic use from 1992 to 2000, in the French community. J Antimicrob Chemother.2004;54(2):524-8.

50. PH I, SG JC, BM P, RP L, LP B, Callens. S. Community-onset extended-spectrum β- lactamase producing Escherichia coli in urinary tract infections in children from 2015 to 2016. Medicine (Baltimore).2017;96(50):8571.

51. Ioanna K, Fani L, Emmanouil A, Maria A,Georgia V. Susceptibility patterns

of uropathogens identified in hospitalized children. Pediatrics International. 2019; 61: 246-51

52. Flammang A, Morello R, Vergnaud M, Brouard J, Eckart P. Étude du profil des résistances bactériennes dansles pyelonephritis of children in 2014. Arch Pediatrics. 2017;24(3):215-24.

53. Tal BN, Shiri NV, Nathan K, Sharon A.Risk analysis of antimicrobial resistance in outpatient urinary tract infections of young healthy adults .J Antimicrobial Chemotherapy.2019;(74) 2:499-502

54. Céire C,Chris M,Andrew L,David M,Alastair DH. Effect of antibiotic prescribing in primary care on antimicrobial resistance in individual patients: systematic review and meta- analysis.BMJ.2010;340:2096.

55. Allen UD, MD N, Fuite L, Chan F, Stephens D. Risk factors for resistance to "first-line" antimicrobials among urinary tract isolates of Escherichia coli in children. CMAJ Can Med Assoc J J Assoc Medicale Can.1999;160(10):1436-40.

Appendix 1:

Information sheet : Urinary tract infections in children

File no.	....	Contact:...............	
Name :	....	First name:...............	
NMS :	....	AGE:.. .<3 months :	YES NO
Gender :	Male		
	Female		

PREVIOUS HOSPITALIZATION FOR IU

- YES

- NO

Urinary tract infection :

- Hautte (PNA)

- Low (cystitis)

Reason for admission :

	Yes	no
- Fever		
- abdominal/lumbar pain		
- low urinary disorders :		
Hematuria.......................		
Pollakiuria.......................		
Urinary burning		
Dysuria		
- digestive disorders :		
diarrhea		
vomiting		

Pathological antecedents :

	NO	YES		
- Immune deficiency (ID)				
- vulvitis				
- intermittent survey				
known uropathy : VUP .... Meguretère............... *RVU .... VNNN .... VN .... SJPU..............	....	....	Antenatal Dg: yes Type:.....................	no
- ancds de PNA			Number :............................. Deadline :.................................	
- ancds explorations (UCR /EUD/Scinti iso)			Deadline:	
- urological surgery ancds :			Type : .... Deadline:.................................	

Antibiotic therapy (ATB) :

	YES	NO
Antibiotic prophylaxis :		
ATB use in the last 3 months :		
ATB use in the last 6 months :		

Clinical status on admission :

	YES	NO
Fever		
- <48 H - > 48 H		
AEG (altered general condition)		
DSH (Dehydration)		
Food tolerance		
Signs of Sepsis:		
EHD alteration chills jaundice		

BIOLOGY

	Yes	No	Value
Hyperleukocytosis			
Hyperleukoneutropenia PNN			
Neutropenia			
Thrombocytopenia			
CRP			
Procalcitonin			
Creatinine			
Clearance Cr			

URINE TEST STRIPS BU :

Nitrites :	
Positive	
Negative	
Leukocyturia	
Positive	
Negative	
Urine appearance :	
Clair	
Disorder	
Purulent	
Thematic	

ECBU :

Preventive antibiotic therapy : Yes No	
Urine collection technique : Middle of the jet Urine collector Bladder probe Suprapubic catheter	
Direct examination:	
GB=.......................... GR =..........................	
Culture : Germ: .... Antibiotic susceptibility testing:................	

Initial antibiotic therapy :

- Combination: 1/ monotherapy

2/ dual therapy

Route :1/ Peros

2/ Intravenous

3/ Intramuscular

- Molecule :1 DOSE (mg/kg/24h) 1- 2- .2-

- Maintained : ☐ ☐ durée :...

- Initial antibitherapy change: ☐☐raison : 1-clinical:......2-antibiogram:......

Relay antibiotic therapy :

- Combination: 1/ monotherapy

2/ dual therapy

- Route :1/ Peros

2/ Intravenous

3/ Intramuscular

- Molecule :1 -DOSE (mg/kg/24h) 1- 2- 2-duration:

Acute phase imaging :

	YES	NO	Results
- Renal ultrasound			Renal abscess: YES/NO
- DMSA scintigraphy			
- URO SCAN			
- URO MRI			

complications :

	YES	NO	
- Renal abscess :			
- Obstructive pleonephrosis :			
- Renal insufficiency :			
- Sepsis :			

DOB :......

AGE:.<3 months : YESNO

Antibiogram :

Germ: ....

Antibiotic name	diameter	Thresholds	Interpreted result Sensitive / intermediate / resistant			CMI
Ampicillin 10ug		14 - 14				
Amoxicillin +ac clavulanique 20-10ug		19- 19				
Amoxicillin +ac clavulanique cystitis		16 - 16				
Ticarcillin 75ug		23 - 23				
Ticarcillin+ ac clavulanique 75-10ug		23 - 23				
Piperacillin 30ug		17 - 20				
Piperacillin +tazobactam 30-6ug		17 - 20				
Cefalexin 30ug		14 - 14				
Mecillinam 10ug		15 - 15				
Cefoxitin 30ug		15 - 19				
Cefuroxime iv30ug		18 - 18				
Cefixime 5ug		17 - 17				
Cefotaxime 5ug		17 - 20				
Ceftazidime 10ug		19 - 22				
Cefepime 30ug		21 - 24				
Azetreonam 30ug		21 - 24				
Ertapenem 10ug						

58

Imipinem 10ug					
Gentamicin 10ug		14 - 17			
Amikacin 30ug		13 - 16			
Netilmicin 10ug		12 - 15			
Tobramycin 10ug		14 - 17			
Nalidixic acid 30ug		14 - 19			
Norfloxacin 10ug		19 - 22			
Ofloxacin 5ug		19 - 22			
Ciproofloxacin 5ug		19 - 22			
Chloramphenicol 30ug		17 -17			
Fosfomycin 200ug		13 - 16			
Tigecycline 15ug		0 - 0			
Nitrofurantoine100ug		11 - 11			
Trimethéoprime+sulfamide 1.25/23.75ug		13 - 16			
Meropeneme (CMI)		0 - 0			
Imipeneme (CMI)		0 - 0			
Ertapeneme (CMI)		0 - 0			
Ciprofloxacin (MIC)		0 - 0			

ANTIBIOTIC RESISTANCE IN URINARY TRACT INFECTION IN CHILDREN

Abstract

Background:

Logistic regression is one of the most widely used statistical analyses in epidemiology to determine risk factors or protective factors for a given disease. The objective of our work was to investigate the usefulness of logistic regression in determining risk factors associated with antibiotic resistance in urinary tract infections (UTI) in children.

Methods :

This was a retrospective and etiological cross-sectional study of a series of children admitted for UTI between January and September 2020.The statistical analysis was bi and then multivariate using binary logistic regression. The results were presented in the form of odds ratios and their confidence intervals.

Results :

A total of 100 bacteriologically documented UTI episodes were included. In univariate analysis the prescription of antibiotics in the previous 3 months was associated with antibiotic resistance with a statistically significant difference for cefuroxime (p= 0.005), cefixime (p= 0.002) and ceftazidime (p= 0.008). In multivariate analysis five factors independently associated with the presence of an extended- spectrum beta-lactamase producing strain were retained in the initial model: previous hospitalization (ORb=3.4, IC95%= [0.92-12.49], p=0.066), malformative uropathy (ORb=3.4, IC95%= [0.92-12.49], p=0.066), recurrence of UTI (ORb=3.16, IC95%=[0.858-11.68],p=0.084), antibiotic use in the previous 3 months (ORb=4.29, IC95%= [1,625-11.355], p=0.003) and age (p=0.332). The Wald-type top-down method concluded to the most parsimonious model containing only the variable previous antibiotic in the previous 3 months (ORa=3.34, IC95%= [1,1-10.18], p=0.002).

Conclusion:

Binary logistic regression allowed us to study the factors associated with antibiotic resistance in UTI in children. Our results underline the need for a therapeutic strategy adapted to our bacterial ecology and targeted actions to address antibiotic resistance factors.

Key-words: Urinary tract infection, Child, Logistic regression, Antibiotic resistance

TABLE OF CONTENTS

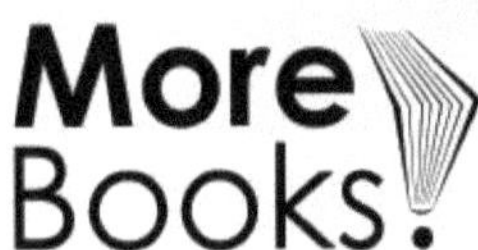

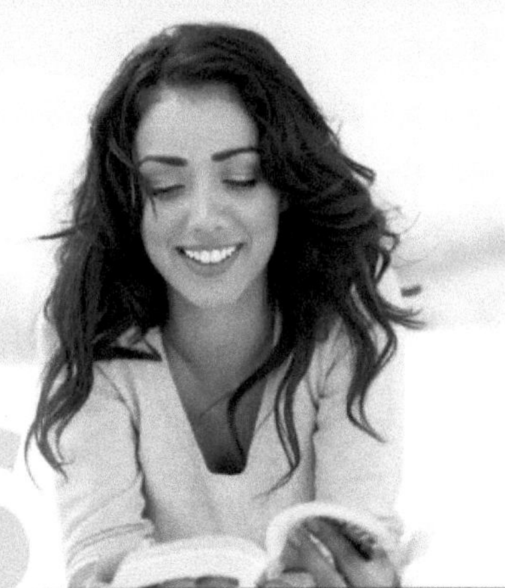

yes I want morebooks!

Buy your books fast and straightforward online - at one of world's fastest growing online book stores! Environmentally sound due to Print-on-Demand technologies.

Buy your books online at
www.morebooks.shop

Kaufen Sie Ihre Bücher schnell und unkompliziert online – auf einer der am schnellsten wachsenden Buchhandelsplattformen weltweit! Dank Print-On-Demand umwelt- und ressourcenschonend produziert.

Bücher schneller online kaufen
www.morebooks.shop

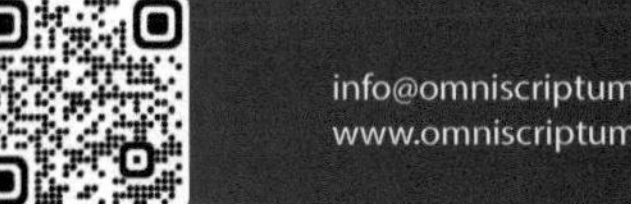

info@omniscriptum.com
www.omniscriptum.com

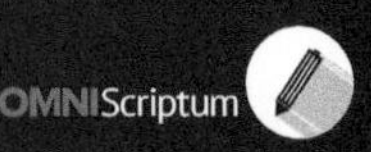

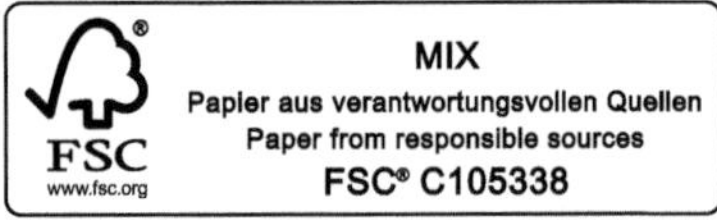

Printed by Books on Demand GmbH, Norderstedt / Germany